CAREERS IN
PRACTICAL NURSING

Licensed Practical Nurse (LPN)

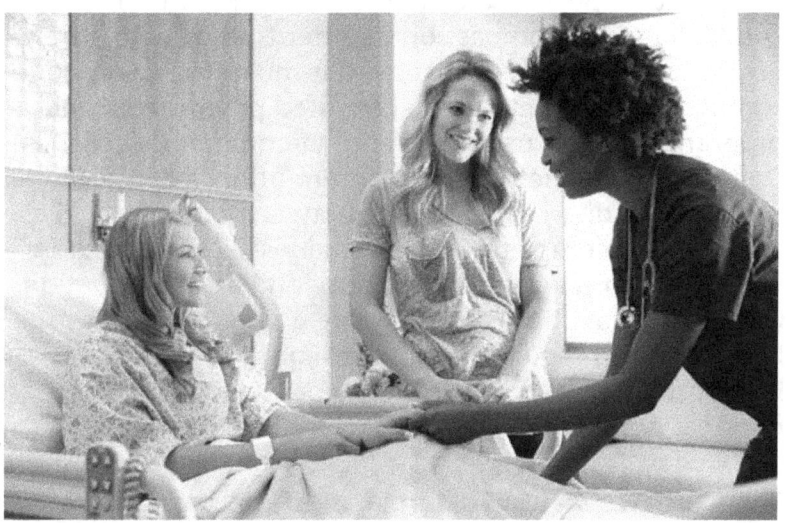

WHEN YOU ARE FEELING AT YOUR WORST, a licensed practical nurse (LPN) is often the first person you see, adding a human touch to a scary medical situation. These healthcare professionals are a vital part of the healthcare system, working under the supervision of doctors and registered nurses (RNs). They provide direct patient care that ranges from feeding and bathing, to checking vital signs and administering medication. In addition to patients are comfortable and well cared for, they keep detailed medical records, monitor patients' conditions, and explain procedures and care plans to patients and family members. In short, the work of LPNs is very similar to that of registered nurses.

LPNS are essential to nursing homes, hospitals, assisted living facilities, rehabilitation centers, and doctors' offices. They also provide one-on-one care in private homes. Most work full time, but part-time jobs are common for those wanting flexibility and more control over their work/life balance.

LPNs need to possess a certain combination of skills, knowledge, and compassion in order to provide the best possible care when patients need it most. The knowledge comes from completing an accredited practical nursing program, which is usually offered at community colleges. Depending on whether the program offers a certificate or an associate degree, it will take between one year and two years to complete. The necessary skills are honed in hands-on clinical experience before and after graduation. Graduates must be licensed before going to work as an LPN. Licensing requirements vary slightly among states, but all states expect applicants to pass a four-part national exam known as the NCLEX.

There are two states, California and Texas that call their licensed nurses "licensed vocational nurses" (LVNs). There is literally no difference between an LPN and an LVN other than where they live and work. They are simply different titles for the same job. The licensing requirements are the same and the duties are the same with only very minor variations. For the purpose of simplicity, the term licensed practical nurse will be used in this report.

In return for a minimal amount of education, you can expect job security and financial stability. There is a serious nursing shortage in the US that is expected to worsen as the Baby Boom population continues to reach retirement age. The nursing shortage may not be good news for those requiring care, but it does mean newly licensed LPNs are assured of good jobs upon graduation. Furthermore, the federal government predicts that there will be continuing demand for LPNs that is far greater than the average for all other occupations. The demand will be greatest in long-term residential care facilities and in home health environments, especially in rural and other medically underserved communities.

While earnings will vary depending on employer and location, the median annual salary for practical nurses is $45,000. The good news is that a growing field with high demand like this is expected to push salaries up significantly over the next 10 years.

Many who choose this career are surprised at the flexibility and choices available to them. LPNs can choose to work for a single employer or rotate through different settings assigned by an agency. They can decide what kinds of patients they care for and even get special certification in certain types of nursing care that will help advance their careers. They can choose their hours and shifts that provide the ideal work/life balance. For the nurse with a yen to move about, traveling nurses are in high demand all over the country. It is a great way to see the country and get paid considerably more than a staff nurse working full time for a single employer.

Make no mistake, nursing is a demanding job, but if you are a compassionate individual with a good tolerance for stress, nothing could be more fulfilling. If you are considering a career in healthcare, becoming a licensed practical nurse could be the right choice for you.

WHAT YOU CAN DO NOW

TO BECOME A PRACTICAL NURSE, you must first graduate from high school. In addition to your graduation requirements, there may be specific course prerequisites for admission to an LPN program. These are usually classes like biology and college level English. Check with the training program you are considering to make sure you have included all prerequisites in your high school curriculum. To get a leg up, take as many Advanced Placement (AP) classes as possible, especially in math and science subjects, and keep your GPA high.

Outside of school, start building your medical skills by taking classes in CPR and first aid. These are commonly offered by community centers, fire departments, and the American Red Cross. Getting these certifications out of the way will take you one step closer to getting your nursing license.

Get some real experience in nursing through volunteer work. Nursing homes, senior centers, and community health centers always need a helping hand. Some hospitals also offer summer volunteer programs for high school students. Volunteering can give you a good idea of what to expect in this career, plus it will add to the weight of your LPN training application and future employment prospects.

Consider joining HOSA-Future Health Professionals, if it is available at your school. This international student organization is recognized by the US Department of Education and by the Association For Career & Technical Education (ACTE). Its mission is to promote career opportunities in the healthcare industry and provide encouragement to all health science students.

HISTORY OF THE CAREER

LONG BEFORE THERE WERE NURSING SCHOOLS and laws regulating the scope of practice, sick and injured members of the community needed caregivers. Historically, those were female friends or family members, until the Dark Ages, when monasteries took on the role of nursing. Nuns and monks continued this tradition until the reformation of the church's role in the Middle Ages. As the church's responsibilities diminished, females convicted of various crimes were compelled to assume nursing duties or face indefinite imprisonment. The mandate continued through outbreaks of the plague, bolstered by the view that if these women died in service it would be no loss to society. However, the nurses discovered and implemented methods and medicines to alleviate the terrible disease, which was eventually eradicated by the end of the 16th century.

The history of licensed practical nursing in the United States begins in the late 1800s. The first formal training program was initiated in 1892 by the YWCA in New York City. Shortly thereafter, the first official school for practical nursing, Ballard School, also opened in New York. The original training covered care for the sick, but also included homemaking skills. It was not until the beginning of the 21st century that education and licensing became formalized, making practical nursing a recognized profession.

World War I created the first serious shortage of practical

nurses. To fill the demand, the Army School of Nursing was formed to help train more nurses, and the Smith Hughes Act provided money for more public practical nursing schools. At the same time, the National League for Nursing developed standards for the scope of practice. Many of the new trainees left nursing after the end of the war. Those who did continue during the 1920s and 1930s worked in public health agencies and as visiting nurses.

A severe nursing shortage arose again during World War II. Training efforts ramped up to produce nurses in accelerated programs focused on the delivery of hands-on nursing care. The desperate need for trained practical nurses prompted the formation of The National Association for Practical Nurse Education and Service (NAPNES) in 1941. Practical nursing students were officially recognized at the 1944 NAPNES conference and shortly after, NAPNES became the first accreditation agency. During the war years, hospitals attracted more workers by offering incentives like monthly stipends, paid tuition, uniforms, housing, and the opportunity to "see the world." In addition to clinics and hospitals, practical nurses were sent on wartime "hardship tours" to North Africa, Europe, and the Pacific. By the end of the war, practical nursing professionals had earned the respect of the general public.

Shortly after World War II, the first licenses for trained practical nurses were issued and national boards of nurse examiners began to emerge. In 1951, the Board of Vocational Nurse Examiners (BVNE) was established. At first, the licenses from this board were granted by waiver, based on experience and physician recommendations. When the first national examinations were instituted in 1952, licenses were no longer granted by waiver and had to be earned. At this time, most training programs were provided in hospitals and licensing was done on the state level. Nursing exams were standardized, but based on each individual state's directive. By 1955, all states had set their own educational standards and regulations for the licensing of practical nurses.

Although practical nursing was becoming firmly established as a profession throughout the 1950s, it was not yet acceptable for women to work outside the home once they married and became mothers. It took the radical 1960s to change attitudes and free women to join the workforce as working wives and mothers.

In the 1970s, it became clear that licensing examinations needed to be standardized nationwide. This realization resulted in the creation of the National Association for Practical Nurse Education and Service (NAPNES) in 1978. In order to ensure public safety, the organization developed the NCLEX-PN examination. It was decided that all practical nurses would have to pass that exam, in addition to completing accredited training.

There is a long history of changes to the practical nurse's role. The foundation of the profession – providing aid and comfort to the sick and injured – has stayed the same since its inception. Since the beginning of the 21st century, the practical aspects of the work have been mostly left up to the policy of the workplace. What a practical nurse can do and is expected to do in a nursing home is different than at a hospital, correctional facility, school, or residence. The role can vary from company to company, too. One nursing home might hire and promote a practical nurse to a head nurse position, while another will only consider an RN for that job. One home health agency might allow a practical nurse to give medications while another does not permit it. This divergence is both a challenge and an opportunity. It can be confusing for new nurses in particular to understand their role, but it also offers versatility and choices.

Although many practical nurses have assumed some of the duties of RNs, it is not precisely known how the role will change in the future. What we do know is there is once again a severe nursing shortage. This time it is not caused by war, but rather an aging population in need of healthcare assistance. The number of practical nurses completing education programs in the US is unlikely to keep pace with the simultaneous decline in supply from retirements and older people filling up nursing homes and assisted living facilities. The LPN is an important entry point into the medical profession and considering the historical need for nurses, their contributions will surely be welcome for the foreseeable future.

WHERE YOU WILL WORK

LICENSED PRACTICAL NURSES ARE VITAL PERSONNEL in hospitals, nursing homes, doctor's offices, and other healthcare facilities. In private and public hospitals, they are typically assigned to work in maternity, surgery, and emergency departments. When considering nursing, most people think of hospitals, but actually fewer than 20 percent of practical nurses work in that environment. There are many more jobs elsewhere.

The largest employer of practical nurses is long-term care facilities. This sector accounts for nearly 40 percent of jobs. It is a broadly defined area that includes nursing homes for the elderly, assisted living facilities, retirement homes, homes for the chronically or mentally ill, hospice services, and rehabilitation services.

Many practical nurses work in the offices of physicians. These offices may be independent, stand-alone practices or associated with clinics, outpatient surgical centers, and urgent care services.

More and more practical nurses can be found working in the home healthcare field where they provide one-on--one, direct private care in patient's residences. Employers in this area include home health agencies, clinic outpatient departments, and niche areas of large medical facilities.

In addition, there are many other settings where practical nurses are employed, such as group homes, schools, military organizations, and correctional facilities.

Work Schedules

Most practical nurses work full time, but this does not necessarily mean working regular business hours. Medical care is needed at all hours of the day. Shifts may be scheduled for nights, weekends, and holidays. In some environments, like hospitals, shifts may be 12 hours on, 12 off, rather than the usual eight hours. There is some flexibility available depending on where you work. Part-time jobs are common. Nearly one out of five practical nurses works part time, and a healthy percentage take temporary assignments, usually through locum tenens agencies.

THE WORK YOU WILL DO

LICENSED PRACTICAL NURSES PROVIDE hands-on basic medical and nursing care to people who are sick, injured, convalescent, or disabled. They are often the first point of contact for patients and their family members, and are therefore the ones who set a positive and reassuring tone for what is to come. The basic goal of the practical nurse is to ensure the comfort of patients by providing essential care that can range from helping patients bathe and eat, to checking vital signs and administering medication. In many cases, the practical nurse is the primary contact for patients. They often answer questions about the healthcare plan and explain procedures. Any change in status is reported to the supervising registered nurse or doctor.

LPNs work under the supervision of a registered nurse or physician. Each state's regulations specify how much supervision is required and what duties a practical nurse is allowed to perform. Every state allows licensed practical nurses to perform a wide variety of functions. On the job, the nurse's daily routine might include any of the following tasks:

- Take vital signs, specifically pulse rate, temperature, respiration rate, and blood pressure

- Compile patient health information and maintain patients' medical records

- Help with dressing, grooming, and personal hygiene

- Change bandages and perform other basic medical treatments

- Administer medication and start IV drips, noting frequency and amounts

- Monitor patient's health and response to medications and other aspects of the care plan

- Set up, clean, and use catheters, oxygen suppliers, and other medical equipment

- Assist doctors and registered nurses with tests and procedures

In some states, experienced licensed practical nurses can assume leadership roles, supervising other practical nurses, nursing assistants and aides, and other unlicensed medical staff.

It is clear that licensed practical nurses handle many of the same types of responsibilities as registered nurses. Both can take and record patient vitals, answer patient questions in person or over the phone, and administer medication that has been prescribed for the patient. In the end, a registered nurse or doctor will have the last word on any medical decision, but the day-to-day work of the practical nurse will often look the same as that of the registered nurse.

Practical nurse training covers a wide variety of healthcare areas, such as emergency care and pediatric nursing, so that the nurses can apply their skills in many areas. For example, feeding and caring for infants are different than feeding and caring for elderly patients with dysphagia or dementia. Whether working in the pediatric department or in a nursing home, licensed practical nurses know how to adjust their skills to provide the most appropriate care.

LPNs work in a variety of settings from hospitals to doctors' offices and everywhere in between. Although the basic skills and duties are similar across the board, the duties will vary depending on the work setting and the state in which they are located.

Hospitals offer a fast-paced environment, divided into many different departments. The most common areas for practical nurses to work in are maternity wards, emergency rooms, and surgical suites. Like all practical nurses, those in hospitals routinely discuss health concerns and issues with patients, care for basic needs like feeding and grooming, and monitor and record patients' status both before and after treatments have taken place. What is different is the level of skill required. Hospitals usually expect licensed practical nurses to perform advanced nursing practices in certain areas under the supervision of a doctor or registered nurse. They are also expected to supervise any nursing aides working within the hospital. It can be an exciting place to work, but can also be challenging and stressful.

A doctor's office is a very different environment from a hospital. It is much quieter and evenly paced. The hours are regular with no night shifts or expectation of being called in on weekends or holidays. Practical nurses working in this setting rarely deal with life-threatening medical conditions. Duties typically involve taking medical histories, preparing patients for examination, giving injections, dressing incisions, and helping with minor surgeries. Orders usually come directly from the doctor rather than from a registered nurse. In some offices, the practical nurse may also be responsible for some administrative tasks, such as making appointments and maintaining medical records.

Unlike hospitals and doctors' offices, nursing facilities provide long-term care to people who are chronically ill, mentally disabled, or in need of rehabilitative services. Some facilities are devoted to the care of the elderly, while others serve the general population. The core duties of the practical nurse in these locations include assessing the health of patients, developing treatment plans, ensuring that rooms are safe and hygienic, supervising nursing aides, and performing administrative work. They may also assist with physical therapy regimes and provide companionship. Basic personal care is essential to the well-being of patients. In these facilities, patients often suffer from ailments that limit their ability to handle simple tasks like dressing themselves or brushing their own teeth. Over time, the nurses become familiar with the patients and their families and it is common for strong relationships to form.

Home healthcare services are a growing work sector for LPNs. Services are often needed by the elderly, but anyone recovering from a serious illness, accident, or surgery is likely to be at home rather than in the hospital. Practical nurses in this sector are usually assigned to individual patients by a private agency. It is the most autonomous situation a practical nurse can have. They work directly with patients and their families under the direction of doctors, but without supervision. The role involves helping patients in their home recover to the point where they are able to care for themselves. Tasks will vary depending on the particular patient, and can include anything from cooking and feeding meals to changing dressings or assisting with physical therapy. Since the patients are often living alone or have limited assistance from friends and family, the practical nurse spends time just talking and offering encouragement. In some cases, they take patients on daily outings. These activities are good for mental health, which is key to fast healing. One of the main responsibilities is to evaluate patient conditions daily and report the status to the doctor.

STORIES OF PRACTICAL NURSES

I Work on a Surgery Team

"I have been an LPN for eight years. My first job after training was in a doctor's office. After a couple of years I was hired by a hospital where I rotated through several departments. After covering for someone in the surgery department, I decided that was where I wanted to be. I got my surgical tech certification and became a permanent member of that department. I was able to handle the certification process while working full time, and the hospital reimbursed me for the costs.

Surgical nursing is a tough field and it can be very stressful. It is also fun because I get to learn something new almost every day. I have mostly the same duties as an RN, except I don't hang blood or push LEDs through IVs.

One of the best features about being a nurse is that you have so many different specialties that you can go into. Nurses do basically the same thing wherever they work so there is no reason to work in an area that doesn't interest you. My advice is to try out different areas to see what gets you excited. I originally had no interest in being in a doctor's office, but I had heard that hospitals would be phasing out LPNs. It turns out that isn't the case since it is cost effective for them to hire an LPN versus an RN. Once I realized I could get a hospital job, I was on my way. I truly enjoy my work now."

I Specialize in Medically Complex and Fragile Pediatrics

"I spend my days working one on one with medically complex children. These are children that require the highest level of care due to their significant chronic conditions. Some have congenital or acquired multisystem diseases, or severe neurologic conditions that cause disabilities. Others are cancer patients or survivors with multiple ongoing disabilities. There are about 3 million of these children in this country. Most need to be cared for in children's hospitals. Some are lucky enough to live at home and go to school – with help. That's where I come in.

I go to school with my patients and tend to their nursing needs throughout the school day and during transportation. I do all the heavy lifting, so to speak, but there is usually a school RN available for advice and support. I also work closely with the parents to make sure we're on the same page. The most challenging part of my job is to keep an upbeat attitude and reassure parents that their precious children are getting the best possible care.

Sometimes it can be difficult knowing where the line is drawn in what I, as an LPN, can legally do and what must be relegated to an RN. There are some tasks the parents can do with their own children, like inflate a g-tube, that I am not permitted to do. A parent can also give their children Tylenol, but I need a physician's order to do that. Something so seemingly simple is often questioned in a home environment.

I had excellent training that was very hands-on clinically. I feel confident in my skills, but I'm continuing my education so I can expand my scope of practice. More education and certifications will allow me to move into case management, which is my goal."

I Care for People with Alzheimer's

"I am the head nurse in an assisted living facility. In my 15 years as an LPN, I have worked in several different kinds of jobs. I started out in a clinic and didn't like it much. Then I moved on to a skilled rehab unit of a long-term care facility where I worked my way up to Coordinator, assessing the functioning capabilities of residents. I loved that job, but it was quite hectic and after 10 years, I decided it was time to slow down.

The work I do now is pretty relaxed by comparison. My typical day starts with giving breakfast and meds to 12 patients. That takes about half an hour. Then I make rounds with doctors, sit in on care-plan meetings, update care plans, and help the director with staffing issues. I am also responsible for auditing charts, and making sure all patient records are up to date on physicals and history. Once a month, there are reports and other paperwork to do. That takes less than an hour and a half total.

At this point in my career, I like the predictable routine and hours. I do work some weekends, but usually my hours are 6:30am to 3:00pm. If I do work on the weekend, I get days off during the week, which is great for getting some personal things done. There isn't much risk of getting burned out because all staff here get 22 vacation days per year. That's an entire month when you figure in the weekends, which aren't counted.

The hardest part of being an LPN, by far, was getting through the training. My advice to aspiring nurses is this: do not underestimate LPN training. It is very, very tough because so much information is concentrated into a small time frame. Be prepared to study into the wee hours and sit for two or three exams every week. There are also clinical shifts four days a week. A lot of people drop out because it's harder than they expected. Be prepared and hang in there. It's hard, but it's worth it. I wouldn't trade my nursing career for anything else."

PERSONAL QUALIFICATIONS

IN ANY MEDICAL SITUATION, THE FIRST PERSON a patient is likely to meet is a practical nurse. That initial interaction is important because it sets the tone for whatever is to follow, whether it is a routine checkup or a major surgery. Because interacting with patients and other healthcare providers is such a big part of their jobs, good interpersonal skills are essential for LPNs. Most choose their profession because they genuinely care about people and are naturally compassionate. The most successful nurses have developed a good bedside manner that puts patients at ease. This isn't always easy. Patients may be scared or have some degree of physical or mental disability that requires extra patience and empathy. Listening carefully and offering emotional comfort can go a long way towards making patients feel better.

Caring for others is a difficult requirement for a nurse, especially if the patient suffers from chronic pain or is in critical condition. Emotional stability is absolutely necessary to avoid succumbing to stress. Emergency situations, varying schedules, and patients' concerned family members can also add to the stress. It is challenging, but practical nurses must be able to maintain composure under the most difficult of circumstances while continuing to provide good care.

All day long, practical nurses are communicating directly with patients, their families, doctors, and other nurses. Solid communications skills are needed to be able to understand and convey important information. For example, they may need to accurately describe a change in a patient's condition to an RN or a physician. Or they may need to carefully explain to a patient what a prescribed medication is and how to administer it when the patient gets home.

A nurse's job is fast paced and often encompasses many different tasks. In many healthcare facilities, there is a shortage of nurses that requires being able to take care of several patients at once. Strong organizational skills are necessary to manage it all without getting frazzled or making mistakes. These skills will help you keep track of patient records, provide pertinent information at a moment's notice, and ensure that each patient receives effective care in a timely manner.

Being detail oriented is also important. Practical nurses are the ones who spend the most time in direct contact with patients. They are expected to notice even the smallest changes in condition, understand the significance of the changes, and convey that information so that patients get the correct care at the right time. Doing so can prevent serious problems from developing and affect future treatment plans. Attention to detail is also key for ensuring that a patient's vitals and medications are correctly recorded each and every time.

Make no mistake – nursing is hard work. It takes a great deal of physical strength and stamina to be on your feet all day, running between patients and supervisors, bending over patients for long periods of time, and moving patients of all shapes and sizes for eight to 12 hours. Practical nurses need to be up to the challenge of performing all tasks with relative ease.

No matter how compassionate and caring you may be, you may not be cut out for working in a medical environment. Are you sure you can tolerate blood, bodily fluids, and all the other smells, sights, and touches that come with treating the human body? It is natural to be a little squeamish, but you cannot let it interfere with your ability to do your job.

ATTRACTIVE FEATURES

NURSING IS A GREAT CAREER CHOICE if you are passionate about helping people. There will be times when you literally save someone's life. That may not happen often, but every single day you will be providing care and comfort to patients in need. Knowing you helped someone can be very gratifying. You will make a difference while doing what you love – caring for others.

Becoming a licensed practical nurse is a great option for getting started in the booming healthcare industry. Unlike most healthcare professions, you can become a nurse without many years of education or training. LPN training programs can get you ready for your first job in less than one year. Better yet, you can prepare to launch a long term, upwardly mobile career in less than two years. By earning an associate degree, you can easily enroll in an LPN-to-RN program while your employer foots the bill.

The job outlook and earning potential for practical nurses are excellent. Once you have received your training, you can be assured there will always be a job available. There is a severe shortage of nurses due to a growing demand for healthcare services. Government statistics indicate that the job growth rate for practical nurses employment is well above the average for all other occupations.

Considering the low entry requirements, the salary and benefits are very good. Many practical nurses earn more money than people with bachelor degrees. The median annual salary for practical nurses is about $50,000, and there are numerous ways to increase income once you get going.

Becoming a practical nurse is an ideal way to be in the healthcare profession while still having a life. Nurses often work full time, but many take advantage of opportunities to work part time, on call, or only accept temporary assignments. If you want to have more time for family, you can take advantage of flexible scheduling. Residential care centers and especially hospitals need to staff nurses around the clock. If you need to look after your kids during the day, for example, you could work a night shift. If being home in time to put dinner on the table is important, you could choose a work setting that has standard business hours, like a physician's office, outpatient clinic, or surgery center. If you want some adventure in your life, traveling nurse jobs are another option. Simply put, a career in practical nursing offers a great work/life balance.

Nursing work can be diverse and interesting. Practical nurses can change paths at any time in their careers. There is a variety of patient care areas to choose from, such as maternity, surgery, or pediatrics. There are also many different settings. You can work in nursing homes, clinics, hospice, home health, private duty, psychiatric, rehab centers, developmental disabilities, assisted living, group homes, and a wide range of other types of healthcare settings. There are additional opportunities outside of direct patient care, like discharge planning, case management, and education. You can also choose an employer like an insurance company, law firm, or school. You can also easily advance your career by becoming an expert through certification programs in specialty areas like oncology, emergency room, labor and delivery, or rehabilitation.

UNATTRACTIVE ASPECTS

NURSING WORK IS HARD, BOTH PHYSICALLY and mentally. Practical nurses are often on their feet for most of the day. They are susceptible to back injuries from lifting and moving patients of all shapes and sizes. There is exposure to all types of germs, viruses, and other pathogens. There is a risk of unwanted chemicals getting into the nose, eyes, or mouth. There is always the possibility of accidental needle sticks during injections. Nurses are taught guidelines for safety and precautions that can prevent such incidents.

The job can be stressful for a variety of reasons. The work can be overwhelming when you are short staffed or there is a sudden influx of new patients to treat. Even ordinary patient loads can create a hectic day that ends in exhaustion. There are also a million details to deal with. Practical nurses are often tasked with keeping notes and updating medical records. There is no room for an overlooked detail or lazy error, no matter how busy the day gets. Incorrect information can have tragic consequences.

Some patients are easy to work with and others are not. Some will appreciate your help and others will add to your stress level. It is important to learn how to relieve stress so that it does not get the better of you.

Once you are on the job, you will notice that you are performing many of the same tasks as your RN counterparts – for less money. The average annual salary of an RN is $75,000, compared to a practical nurse's salary of $50,000. It only makes sense that the salary of an entry-level practical nurse would be less than that of an RN. It takes much less time to get trained. In order to reduce the amount of time it takes to get trained and into your first job, you will have to compromise the amount you can earn. Your income will increase as time goes on, but after a couple of years, many practical nurses start thinking about going back to school to become an RN. That plan is sensible and can work well for your long-term career goals.

Hospitals and nursing homes need nurses around the clock. You may have to work varied shifts including nights, weekends, and holidays. There are positions that offer 9 to 5, Monday through Friday scheduling, but they sometimes pay less and there are fewer opportunities for advancement.

If you are repulsed by the sight and smell of blood and other bodily fluids, nursing is probably not your best career choice. Nurses often deal with blood and other bodily fluids, particularly in a hospital setting.

EDUCATION AND TRAINING

A COLLEGE DEGREE IS NOT NECESSARY to become a licensed practical nurse. However, training from an accredited school is required. Contact your state board of nursing for a list of approved programs near you. An approved educational program that leads to a non-degree certificate takes about a year to complete. This kind of program is commonly offered by technical schools, community colleges, and even some high schools and hospitals. Applicants must have a high school diploma or equivalent, and in some cases, there is an entrance exam.

It is tempting to go the shortest route possible, but it is much better to earn an associate degree. An Associate Degree in Nursing (AND), which usually takes six to 12 additional months, provides a solid career foundation for the long run. It is also a higher credential that demonstrates to employers you have greater knowledge and skills. More importantly, if you want to advance your career and become a registered nurse (RN) at any point, having an associate degree will make the leap much easier. Instead of starting from scratch, you can enroll in an LPN-to-RN program, where your LPN course credits will shorten the time commitment. Many nurses with an AND take an entry-level position and then use employer-provided tuition reimbursement programs to complete their training to become an RN.

Programs are available from most community colleges as well as state colleges and universities. In addition to a high school diploma or GED, there are often certain prerequisite courses required for admission. High school students are advised to check with the school of their choice well before their senior year to make sure those courses are completed.

Programs cover medical topics, plus general education core subjects. Classroom learning includes courses in anatomy and physiology, biology, pharmacology, nutrition, chemistry, microbiology, and other nursing subjects. There are also elective courses in specialized areas like emergency care, surgical nursing, pediatrics, obstetrics, and geriatrics. These courses can provide the foundation for specialization certification. Most programs also include nursing license preparation, which is a recap of the program combined with preparation for state licensing examinations.

All programs include hands-on training in a clinical setting. This is usually formal supervised training in a nearby hospital. It allows nursing students to gain valuable experience and may also lead to possible job offers upon graduation. In addition, most programs either offer or require participation in internship programs.

Online Programs

Some community colleges and vocational schools offer LPN programs online. However, these programs are never fully online. The skills that nurses need can only be learned in a clinical environment. Therefore, if you enroll in an online program, you will most likely do your clinical work at a local hospital coordinated with the school, where you will learn how to actually provide nursing to real patients and work within a medical team.

Licensing and Certification

All LPNs and LVNs must have a license. After completing your training program, you need to take the National Council Licensure Examination (NCLEX). Since each state has different eligibility criteria, you will need to check with your state board of nursing to ensure you have met the requirements in order to take the exam. There are testing sites located all over the country, but before scheduling your exam you will need to first apply for "Authorization to Test" through your local board of nursing and with the National Council of State Boards of Nursing. Spots tend to fill up fast, so you should get signed up as soon as possible. Just make sure you allow yourself plenty of time to study.

The NCLEX exam covers four areas:

Safe, effective care environment, including infection control

Psychosocial integrity, including coping and adaptation skills

Health promotion and maintenance, including development through the lifespan, health problem prevention methods, and early detection of disease

Physiology integrity, including basic care and comfort, pharmacological and parenteral therapies, and reduction of risk.

There are also some professional certifications that can demonstrate extensive knowledge in a certain area. These certifications show that a nurse has advanced knowledge and skills in a specialized area. Some of the most popular certifications are:

- Patient counseling certification
- IV certification
- Advanced life support certification
- Long-term and hospice care certification

EARNINGS

THE MEDIAN ANNUAL SALARY FOR practical nurses is about $50,000. The lowest 10 percent earn less than $35,000, and the highest 10 percent earn more than $65,000. In some circumstances, the median rises to more than $55,000. This does not include bonuses, overtime, holiday pay, and other benefits. Full-time positions typically come with holiday pay and paid sick time. Depending on the healthcare facility, there may also be opportunities to earn bonuses and enroll in profit sharing programs.

Salaries differ according to what area of the healthcare system you are working in. For example, the National Federation of Licensed Practical Nurses reports that large city medical centers will generally pay a higher salary than local community hospitals in smaller towns. Government facilities like VA hospitals pay the most, around $60,000 on average. This is followed closely by nursing and residential care facilities. Home healthcare, which has historically been a notoriously low-paying field, has lately been required to raise wages due to the extreme shortage of qualified nurses. Pay is now on par with all nursing positions across the board.

The lowest pay, $40,000 on average, goes to nurses working in the offices of physicians. Traveling nurses working for locum tenens agencies earn about $45,000 a year from wages, but the actual compensation is considerably higher. There is usually extra compensation to help cover the expense of travel and housing.

Pay and benefits will vary even more by geographic location. The highest earnings, $60,000 and up, are found on both coasts and in the western states of Nevada, California, Alaska, and Arizona. New York, Oregon, Washington, Colorado, New Mexico, Delaware, and New Hampshire are not far behind. In the lower Midwest, and in most Southern states, nurses earn about $40,000. The rest – mostly the upper Midwest, Texas, Florida, Utah, Wyoming, Maine, and Vermont – are in the $35,000 to $40,000 range. You will notice that in most cases, salaries are fairly closely tied to the cost of living so it is questionable if there is any advantage in relocating to a higher paying state.

Although licensed practical nurses do not top the pay scale of nursing jobs, there are ways to improve earnings. The best way is to get the necessary training and degree to become a registered nurse. Certain employers, especially hospitals, will offer financial help with the cost of doing this.

Another way to boost employability and make yourself more valuable is to obtain a professional certification in a specialized area. For example, the popular IV certification or advanced life support certification can easily boost income by 20 percent or more.

A quick and simple way to increase your paycheck is to volunteer for available overtime. Depending on whether it is a weekday, weekend, or holiday, that can mean earning 1.5 or two times the normal salary. It may be tiring working those extra hours, but the overtime pay adds up quickly.

OPPORTUNITIES

THERE ARE APPROXIMATELY 725,000 practical nursing jobs in the US today. As the nursing shortage continues to worsen, the number of jobs opening up is forecast to experience double digit growth in the near term. In most areas of the country, the job growth rate is much faster than average for all other occupations. One reason for the good job outlook is the large number of practical nurses that will be retiring. In fact, most of the current practical nurses are nearing the retiring phase of their life. This means that for the foreseeable future, there will continue to be a great need for newly trained nurses to fill the vacancies.

Aging within the general population is another huge factor contributing to the nursing shortage. Every day now, roughly 10,000 Baby Boomers are turning 65 years old. This rate of aging will continue until the year 2030. As people get older, they naturally require more medical attention. People are living longer and the longer they live, the more likely they will experience chronic health problems. As a result, practical nurses are very much in demand to care for older Americans, especially in long term care environments. This includes residential care facilities (nursing homes), assisted living facilities, and home health care. The demand for practical nurses in long term care facilities is expected to increase by 30 percent over the next few years. The growth rate is even higher for home health care services. This is primarily due to technological advances that allow many people to avoid long hospital stays and instead recover at home.

New practical nurses will find the least competition for a job in rural and other medically underserved areas. Hospitals and other 24/7 facilities need practical nurses around the clock, even on weekends and holidays. Since this may not be appealing to some job seekers, competition for those shifts is often less intense. On the other hand, jobs in outpatient care centers and physicians' offices attract many applicants because they offer regular weekday hours and a comfortable workplace environment.

Practical nurses who want to advance their careers have several good choices. The most common is getting the necessary education and training to become an RN. That typically translates into more job responsibilities and higher pay. Another gateway to career advancement is to obtain certification in a specialty area. Candidates with certification in gerontology or intravenous (IV) therapy are in high demand. The highest growth rate of all for practical nurses is in the hospice area. Licensed practical nurses with certification in hospice care will have the best chance of receiving offers from multiple employers.

The one area where the hiring of practical nurses has slowed is in hospitals. While there will always be a need for their services, the demand is expected to lessen over time as more outpatient procedures occur or treatment is done in a doctor's office and patients recover at home.

GETTING STARTED

THE NEED FOR LICENSED PRACTICAL NURSES has never been greater. Once you have your training and get your LPN license, there will certainly be a job waiting for you. Actually there will be many opportunities to consider. To make sure you can land the job you want the first time out in the workforce, there are things you can do to impress prospective employers.

Since this will likely be your first job out of high school, your résumé will be a little skinny. There is much you can do to fill it up with relevant skills and experience. There are numerous student nursing internships available and most of them pay very well. It is a good idea to intern in several different areas to get a good sense of where you would like to practice nursing once you are licensed.

While you are waiting to be admitted to an internship program, get experience by volunteering. Nursing homes and assisted living centers are especially open to volunteers with some nursing education, even if it is just a few months. Make sure you have your CPR (Cardiopulmonary Resuscitation) and AED (Automated External Defibrillator) certifications before applying to internships or volunteer positions. These are widely available, at low cost, including from your local Red Cross.

Start right away to build a network of contacts and

gather letters of recommendation. There are many ways to find job openings, but most nurses find the best jobs through their contacts. Your network can start with supervisors and teachers, but do not stop there. Join professional nursing associations and attend their conferences. Meet recruiters at job fairs, join student nursing groups at school, and volunteer or get a part-time job at a hospital. Every situation that puts you in contact with potential employers is an opportunity to make an impression and to make your ambitions known.

Job openings are posted in many places. Start with your school. Your counselor will show you where to find notices of job openings and job fairs. Check those regularly so you are first in line to get interviewed.

Next, go online. The big, general job sites like GlassDoor and Indeed will have nursing jobs posted. Rather than sort through thousands of jobs of all kinds, focus on the many sites devoted to the nursing field such as NursingJobs.com, IHireNursing.com, and NurseRecruiter.com. These sites will make your job search a breeze. You can search by license type, state, and area of interest. Professional nursing associations also post jobs on their websites.

If you are not sure what kind of nursing you want to do or feel you need more experience to get into the kind of job you want, consider working for a Locum Tenens agency. There are many of these agencies that are devoted to providing temporary placements for nurses of all levels. You can start making money immediately, even as a beginner. Practical nurses are needed everywhere, so as an LPN you also have the opportunity to travel to places you would like to see. Traveling nurses usually receive stipends for travel and housing expenses in addition to the salary. Contracts can be as short as a couple of weeks or as long as a year. They are usually around three months long. You can choose how long you want to work and whether you want to be available part time or full time.

ASSOCIATIONS

■ **Association For Career and Technical Education**
https://www.acteonline.org

■ **National Association of Licensed Practical Nurses**
http://nalpn.org

■ **National Council of State Boards of Nursing**
https://www.ncsbn.org

■ **National Federation of Licensed Practical Nurses**
http://www.nflpn.org

■ **National Association for Practical Nurse Education and Service (NAPNES)**
https://napnes.org

■ **American Nurses Association**
https://www.nursingworld.org

WEBSITES

■ **Nurse Jobs**
https://nurse.org/jobs

■ **Nursing Jobs**
Nursingjobs.com

■ **I Hire Nursing**
Ihirenursing.com

■ **Nurse Recruiter**
Nurserecruiter.com

Copyright 2019
Institute For Career Research
CAREERS INTERNET DATABASE

www.careers-internet.org

www.ingramcontent.com/pod-product-compliance
Lightning Source LLC
Chambersburg PA
CBHW071200220526
45468CB00003B/1102